Vegan Diet

A Stir Fry Cookbook with 70 Delicious Vegetarian Recipes

(A Quick & Easy cookbook for beginners)

Johnie Burder

Published by Robert Satterfield Publishing House

© Johnie Burder

All Rights Reserved

Vegan Diet Cookbook: A Stir Fry Cookbook with 70 Delicious Vegetarian Recipes (A Quick & Easy cookbook for beginners)

ISBN 978-1-989787-11-3

All rights reserved. No part of this guide may be reproduced in any form without permission in writing from the publisher except in the case of brief quotations embodied in critical articles or reviews.

Legal & Disclaimer

The information contained in this book is not designed to replace or take the place of any form of medicine or professional medical advice. The information in this book has been provided for educational and entertainment purposes only.

The information contained in this book has been compiled from sources deemed reliable, and it is accurate to the best of the Author's knowledge; however, the Author cannot guarantee its accuracy and validity and cannot be held liable for any errors or omissions. Changes are periodically made to this book. You must consult your doctor or get professional medical advice before using any of the suggested remedies, techniques, or information in this book.

TABLE OF CONTENT

Part 1 1

Introduction.. 2

Vegan Sausage.. 2

Vegan Ground Nut Pizza.. 4

Buckwheat With Stuffing....................................... 6

Vegan Sandwich With Avocado And Radish.......... 7

Pumpkin Naan 8

Pancake With Fruit Sauce..................................... 10

Lenten Banana Pancakes...................................... 11

Bread With Zucchini And Spices 13

Vegetable Rolls 14

Waffles Falafel 17

Vegan Casserole From Carrots 18

Roll With Chickpeas... 19

Movie Clips 21

Cecina 23

Bean Hummus 24

Vegetarian Rice Pie Bath-Ching 25

Falafel 27

Chile 28

Manty With Pumpkin, Cabbage And Potatoes 30

Curry 32

Lemon Rice 34

Bulgur With Spinach 35

Omelet From Chickpea Flour With Tomato 37

Vegetables In The Oven 39

Stew With Tofu 41

Burger Vegan 43

Chile Con 47

Manti With Mushrooms And Lentils 49

The Vegan Velininge 50

Cabbage Rolls 54

Stewed Soybean "Meat" 57

Curry With Eggplant And Chickpeas 59

Potatoes With Mushrooms 61

Bulgur With Green Peas 62

Eggplant - Steak With Celery Puree 64

Chickpeas In Tomato Sauce 67

Spinach With Mushrooms 70

Pasta With Homemade Tomato Sauce 71

Eggplant With Coconut Milk 73

Vegan Shakshuka 74

Pancakes With Zucchini And Sauce 76

Vegetable Stew In Provençal 77

Part 2 79

Introduction 80

STEP 1: KNOW THE HISTORY OF THE VEGAN MOVEMENT 81

STEP 2: PLAN THE SHIFT INTO BEING A VEGAN 84

STEP 3: MAKE SMALL CHANGES 86

STEP 4: DO IT RIGHT - LEARN ABOUT VEGAN NUTRITION 88

STEP 5: LEARN AS MUCH AS YOU CAN ABOUT THE BENEFITS OF BEING A VEGAN 91

STEP 6: LOOK AT THE LIVES OF OTHER VEGANS 95

Start It Right 96

STEP 7: VISIT A DOCTOR 97

STEP 8: COMMIT TO A VEGAN LIFESTYLE 99

STEP 9: TELL YOUR FAMILY AND CLOSE FRIENDS 100

STEP 10: WEAN OFF ON EGGS 102

STEP 11: WEAN OFF ON MILK AND DAIRY 104

STEP 12: BE FAMILIAR WITH VEGETABLES 106

- Step 13: Research On Vegetable Recipes............................... 108
- Step 14: Know Your Fruits 110
- Step 15: Research On Fruit Recipes 112
- Step 16: Look For Other Protein Sources - Soy 113
- Step 17: Look For Other Proteins Sources Apart From Soy 115
- Eating And Cooking Vegan Good 117
- Step 19: Look For Vegan Versions Of Your Favorite Food .. 119
- Step 20: Plan Your Vegan Menu.. 121
- Step 21: Look For Places To Shop For Vegan Ingredients.... 123
- Step 22: Shop For Vegan Ingredients 125
- Step 23: Cook And Be Adventurous 127
- Step 24: Take The Right Supplements 128
- Step 25:Try Out Vegan Restaurants..................................... 130
- Step 26: Share Your Lifestyle.. 132
- Step 27: Get Rid Of Other Animal-Based Products 133

STEP 28: JOIN A SUPPORT GROUP	135
Sustaining The Vegan Lifestyle	135
STEP 29: KEEP LEARNING	136
STEP 30: REMEMBER WHY	137
STEP 31: DON'T GIVE UP	138
About The Author	139

Part 1

Introduction

Veganism is considered a more severe form of vegetarianism. It implies a complete refusal to eat food of animal origin. From the diet are excluded: milk, cheese, butter, sour-milk products and, of course, eggs. But the vegan menu remains diverse! There is a huge amount of vegan recipes, which are also called lean. This book is suitable for everyone!

Vegan sausage

Ingredients:

- Yellow peas - 1 glass

- Water - 3 glasses
- Vegetable oil - 50 g
- Beetroot - 1 piece
- Coriander - 1 teaspoon
- Nutmeg - 0.5 teaspoon
- Salt - 1 teaspoon
- Ground pepper - 0.5 teaspoon
- Dried marjoram - 0.5 teaspoon

Preparation:

1. Peas and rinse for several minutes in a frying pan. Then grind into dust in a coffee grinder. Pour the resulting flour with hot water. Within seven minutes, cook the resulting pea mass until it is completely ready, and then leave it to cool off for a short while somewhere in

a cool place. And while the raw beetroot is rubbed on a small grater, squeeze out the juice from it, enough 1 tablespoon.

2. Add spices and salt to the cooled pea puree. Mix in a blender until smooth. Add beet juice, butter, if necessary, spices and salt, whisk again.

3. The resulting mass is put in a mold; you can use a plastic bottle, cutting it from one end. Leave in the refrigerator for the night.

Vegan ground nut pizza

Ingredients:

- Wheat flour - 1/2 cup
- Water - 125 ml

- Olive oil - 2 tablespoons
- Provencal herbs - 1/2 teaspoon
- Salt and black pepper
- Champignons - 4 pieces
- Zucchini - 1/6 pcs.
- Olives - 2-3 pieces
- Tomatoes - 1 piece

Preparation:

Combine all the ingredients for the cake and let stand for 30 minutes. Lubricate the frying pan with olive oil and spread the dough. Put in the oven at 220 sleeps for 10-15 minutes. The cake should brown and easily leave the frying pan. Zucchini, mushrooms and tomatoes cut very thinly, olives on quarters. Lie in layers on the finished cake and again put in the oven for another 10-15 minutes.

Buckwheat with stuffing

Ingredients:

- Buckwheat flour - 450 g
- Wheat flour - 50 g
- Salt - 1 teaspoon
- Cumin - 1 teaspoon
- Water - 380 ml
- Potatoes - 3-4 pieces
- Cauliflower - 150 g
- Bulgarian pepper - 1/4 pieces
- Salt - 3/4 teaspoon, black pepper, chili flakes

- Cilantro

Preparation:

Of all the ingredients knead the dough. Cover it with a damp towel and leave for 30 minutes. Boil the potatoes until cooked in boiling salted water. Then strain and mash. Cut the cabbage in a blender. Pepper chops finely. Add to the potato along with the rest of the ingredients of the filling and mix. The dough is divided into 6 parts and rolled each into a circle. Put the stuffing. Protect the edges towards the center. Slightly roll out the rolling pin. Fry on both sides in a dry hot frying pan.

Vegan sandwich with avocado and radish

Ingredients:

- Unleavened bread - 4-6 slices
- Avocado - 1 piece
- Radish - 4-6 pieces
- Micro green sprouts or any greens

Preparation:

Avocado with a fork. Greens if necessary cut. Cut the radish into thin slices. Smear on the puree of avocado bread, put a slice of radish and sprinkle with herbs. You can cut it in half for convenience.

Pumpkin Naan

Ingredients:

- Flour - 2 cups
- Bitten pumpkin - 1 glass
- Green - a beam
- Salt, spices
- Vegetable oil
- Cilantro - bundle
- Lemon juice - 1-2 teaspoon
- Salt, water, ginger

Preparation:

Mix in the bowl all the ingredients for the dough, knead to a homogeneous consistency. Sprinkle the table with flour, pinching off the pieces to roll them in the form of round cakes. Bake in a dry frying pan on both sides. Ingredients for the sauce grind in a blender. Serve cakes with hot sauce.

Pancake with fruit sauce

Ingredients:

- Wheat flour - 1 glass
- Oatmeal flour - 1 glass
- Mineral water with gas - 2.5 glasses
- Salt
- Vegetable oil
- Bananas - 2 pieces
- Dates - 4-6 pieces
- Dried apricots or prunes - 4-6 pieces

Preparation:

Flour sifts through a sieve, mineral water, a tablespoon of vegetable oil and mix the salt to a homogeneous mass with a blender. To make the dough well mixed, the mineral water should be a little warm. Well grease the frying pan with vegetable oil and fry pancakes on both sides. Dried fruits for an hour or longer soak in warm water, then rinse well. For banana sauce, mix bananas, dried apricots and dates in a blender.

Lenten banana pancakes

Ingredients:

- Wheat flour - 1 glass

- Buckwheat flour - 1/2 cup
- Oat bran - 1/2 cup
- Vegetable oil - 2 tablespoons
- Banana - 2 pieces
- Water - 2 1/2 cups
- Salt, vanilla

Preparation:

Bananas and water are turned into a homogeneous puree in a blender. Add all the remaining ingredients to it and mix thoroughly until smooth. The dough should get thicker than usual. Fry such pancakes on a Teflon pan without oil. The frying pan should be warmed up and spread the scoop on the surface evenly. Fry on both sides, gently turning, as the dough is not very plastic.

Bread with zucchini and spices

Ingredients:

- Zucchini - 1 piece
- Flour whole-grain flour - 2 cups
- Olive oil - 1/2 cup
- Cilantro - 1 bundle
- Zira - 1 teaspoon
- Coriander - 1/2 teaspoon
- Turmeric - 1 teaspoon

Preparation:

Grate the zucchini on a fine grater, add flour, spices, olive oil and mix well. Roll out the thin burrs. Dry in a dry frying pan for a minute on each side.

Vegetable rolls

Ingredients:

- Frozen vegetable mixture - 1 kg
- Breadcrumbs - 80 g
- Parsley - 5-6 branches
- Olive oil - 4 tablespoons
- Salt, freshly ground black pepper
- Rukkola - 1 large bunch
- Olive oil - 4 tablespoons
- Flour - 1 glass
- Vegetable oil - 3 tablespoons

Preparation:

Knead the dough from flour, a pinch of salt, butter and 2 tablespoons of warm water. Turn it into a film and leave it for 1 hour. Pour into the frying pan 4 tablespoons oil and lay out the frozen vegetables, pour in 1/2 cup of hot water and simmer under the lid over medium heat for 10 minutes. Then remove the lid, season with salt and pepper, allow the remaining liquid to evaporate. Grind in a blender bread crumbs and parsley; mix with stewed vegetables, pepper and salt. Roll out the dough on a sheet of parchment, and then very gently stretch it with your hands to make the dough thin. Put the vegetables on the dough, leaving 3 cm on each edge, and wrap them inside, on the filling. Collapse the roll, oil and bake in a preheated oven for 200 ° C for 30 minutes. For cream at the arugula remove the stems, crush the leaves with butter until a smooth creamy state, salt to taste. Strudel cut into slices, serve portionwise, watering sauce.

Waffles falafel

Ingredients:

- Boiled chickpeas - 3 cups
- Flour - 2-3 tablespoons
- Vegetable oil - 1 tablespoon
- Pepper, turmeric, cumin, coriander, salt
- Ground flax - 1 teaspoon
- Parsley or coriander - 1/2 beam

Preparation:

In a blender, grind all the ingredients to a homogeneous consistency. Warm up the waffle iron, oil it and cook waffles, until golden brown. Serve with your favorite sauces.

Vegan casserole from carrots

Ingredients:

- Carrots - 450 g
- Sunflower seeds - 150 g
- Pumpkin seeds - 150 g
- Parsley - 1 tablespoon
- Rosemary - 0.5 teaspoon
- Vegetable oil and salt

Preparation:

Carrots boil, cool and clean, curtain. Seeds are ground in a blender or coffee grinder. In the ground seeds add rosemary, chopped parsley. Mix the carrot puree and a mixture of seeds, salt to taste. The form for baking slightly oiled put the mixture and very tightly tampers. Heat the oven to 200 ° C, and send there the filled form. Depending on the thickness of the casserole, the time will be from 25 to 40 minutes until crisp. The thicker it will be, the more juicy inside - count to taste.

Roll with chickpeas

Ingredients:

- Nut - 1 glass
- Cilantro - 1/4 cup

- Lavash - 4-6 leaves
- Salad leaves - 4-6 pieces
- Tomato - 1-2 pieces
- Raw cashews - 1 glass
- Lime juice - 1 tablespoon
- Hot peppers - 1 piece
- Fragrant pepper - 1 teaspoon
- Ginger - 1 teaspoon
- Cinnamon - 1/2 teaspoon
- Dried thyme - 1/2 teaspoon
- Black pepper - 1/4 teaspoon
- Water - 2-4 tablespoon
- Salt

Preparation:

For cashew sauce pre-soak for 30 minutes, then drain and rinse the water. Mix all the ingredients for the sauce with a blender until smooth. Chickpea dunk for the night, boil. Cilantro chops. Cut the tomatoes into slices. To collect rolls, spread the sauce on the pita bread sheets, lay out lettuce leaves, tomato slices, chickpeas, coriander, wrap tight and serve.

Movie clips

Ingredients:

- Kinoa - 1 glass
- Vegetable broth - 2 glasses

- Crushed almonds - 1 tablespoon
- Crushed sunflower seeds - 1 tablespoon
- Cucumber - 1 piece
- Carrots - 1/2 pieces
- Avocado - 1/4 pcs.
- Nori sheets - 4 pieces

Preparation:

Rinse the movie, put in a saucepan, add two cups of broth and put on fire. Bring to a boil and lower the heat, cook the rump for 15 minutes. Drain excess liquid; add almonds and seeds, mix. Cool it down. Cut into thin strips of cucumber, peeled carrot, and avocado. Put the food film on the table, and the nori sheet on it. Distribute the film over the entire surface, retreating one centimeter from the top edge. Put the vegetables on the opposite edge. Twist the roll. Before serving rolls, cut them into pieces two centimeters thick.

Cecina

Ingredients:

- Nut flour - 1 glass
- Water - 1,5 glasses
- Olive oil - 2 tablespoons
- Salt pepper

Preparation:

Heat oven to 230 ° C. Pour the water into a bowl and slowly stir the chickpea flour.

Add salt and pepper. Let stand at room temperature for as long as possible. Heat the cast-iron frying pan over medium-high heat. Add 2 tablespoons. olive oil, pour into it a chutney mixture and hold on the fire for 30-60 seconds. Do not turn. Put in a hot oven for about 25 minutes. The edges should be roasted to a light crust, and the color should be changed to light golden.

Bean hummus

Ingredients:

- White beans - 1 pot
- Olive oil - 3 tablespoons
- Dill - bundle
- Lemon juice - 3 tablespoons

- Salt, spices

Preparation:

Mix all ingredients in a blender until smooth. Beans can be prepared in advance. Ready to serve hummus, sprinkled with herbs with olives, carrots, cucumbers and other sliced vegetables.

Vegetarian rice pie bath-ching

Ingredients:

- Leaves of Savoy cabbage - 10 pieces
- Rice - 500 g
- Peas frozen green - 300 g
- Tofu - 250 g

- Broccoli 250 g
- Salt, spices

Preparation:

1. Rinse rice and soak in cold water for 8-10 hours. Then rinse again, dry, salt.
2. Tofu and broccoli to grind separately and combine with spices, salt.
3. Peas defrost, grind, salt.
4. Cut cabbage on leaves, turn over with boiling water. All the ingredients are divided into ten parts for five pies, a mixture of tofu-broccoli in five parts. Add two leaves together, put rice on top (50 g) Then a layer of peas, top with a layer of broccoli and tofu. Again peas and rice again. Each layer should be well sealed in hands before laying out.

5. Then wrap in the leaves, forming an envelope with even sides. Wrap with foil.

6. Put pies on the bottom of a deep pan, pour boiling water, cover and cook for about 1 hour until rice and cabbage are ready.

Falafel

Ingredients:

- Nut - 1 glass
- Lemon juice - 3 tablespoons
- Cilantro and parsley - bundle
- Flax - ¼ cup
- Breadcrumbs - ¼ cup
- Salt, spices

- Olive oil

Preparation:

Chick the duck for the night, rinse and boil until done. Mix chickpeas, lemon juice, herbs, salt and spices in a blender. Flax grind and mix with breadcrumbs. Form small balls, tightly squeezing the resulting mixture and roll in breadcrumbs. Fry in a frying pan in oil until golden brown. Serve with fresh salad and sauces.

Chile

Ingredients:

- Celery - 2-3 stems
- Red pepper bulgarian - 1 piece
- Spicy green pepper - 1 piece

- Tomatoes - 4-5 pieces
- Vegetable broth - 1-2 glasses
- Beans ready - 1 glass
- Ready-to-eat beans - 1 glass
- Chile, cumin, oregano, pepper, salt
- Olive oil

Preparation:

1. Vegetables peeled and cut into small pieces. In a deep frying pan fry the hot pepper, celery, bell pepper, then add chopped tomatoes, broth. Add beans, beans, spices and cook for another 10-15 minutes.

2. Serve with cashew sour cream and herbs.

Manty with pumpkin, cabbage and potatoes

Ingredients:

- Water - 200 ml
- Flour 400 - 450 g
- Salt - ½ teaspoon
- Vegetable oil - 25 ml
- Potatoes - 300 g
- Pumpkin - 300 g
- Cabbage - 150 g
- Salt - to taste
- Vegetable oil - 1-2 tablespoons
- Black pepper powder, zeira

Preparation:

1. Dough. In a measuring beaker, mix 200 ml of water, salt and 25 ml of vegetable oil. Sift flour, pour into the bowl "well" - with a hole in the middle, there to pour water and oil. First, knead with a fork, stirring in a circle, gradually taking flour from the edges. When the dough becomes thick, knead with your hands. Tight dough should be wrapped in a package / food film and give a "rest" 20 minutes in the refrigerator. While the dough is resting, make a stuffing. All components of the filling are cut into small cubes of approximately the same size. Add to taste black pepper, seasoning, a couple of spoons of vegetable oil, and stir.

2. You can make manty. Make a dough out of the dough and cut into slices the size of a large walnut. Roll out thinly.

For each pancake, put a full tablespoon of the filling.

3. To blind manties: alternately to connect-blind the middle of opposite edges, for example, first "top and bottom", and then the right and left edges. If you cook manti in water, and not steamed, then do not leave holes, well sealing the edges of the dough. So that the mantles are not stuck to the steamer, you need to oil the grate with oil, put manties on it and cook for 15-20 minutes.

Curry

Ingredients:

- Vegetables - 700 g
- Soya pieces - 200 g
- Almond - 100 g

- Coconut milk - 250 ml
- Ginger root - 1 cm
- Coriander - 1 teaspoon
- Saffron - 1 teaspoon
- Turmeric - 1 teaspoon
- Pepper spicy - 1 teaspoon
- Vegetable oil - 6 tablespoon
- Green - 1 beam

Preparation:

Vegetables can be used frozen, the composition of the mixture of your choice. Soya pieces boil according to the instructions on the package. In a spoon of vegetable oil fry the mixture of spices for 15 minutes, stirring constantly. Cut the vegetables into pieces of the same size, mix. Separately fry thinly sliced ginger. Add spices and almonds to it, simmer for another 5 minutes. In a separate frying pan, simmer the vegetable mixture. Transfer vegetables to spices and ginger, add soya slices, coconut milk and simmer for 15 minutes. Serve the dish hot. Decorate with chopped herbs.

Lemon rice

Ingredients:

- Rice - 1 glass
- Water - 2 glasses
- Vegetable oil - 2 tablespoons
- Lemon juice - 1/3 cup
- Spices - turmeric, curry, cumin

- Parsley greens - to taste

Preparation:

Rice to wash and soak for 10-15 minutes, then drain the water. Meanwhile, heat the oil in a saucepan, add the spices. After 1-2 minutes, set the pan off fire and allow the oil to cool. In the pan add rice and mix with spices and butter, add 2 cups of water. Cook for 25 minutes. After adding lemon juice and herbs, stir, cook for 5 more minutes or let stand for 5-10 minutes.

Bulgur with spinach

Ingredients:

- Bulgur - 1 glass

- Water - 1 1/2 cups
- Fresh spinach - 150 g
- Vegetable oil - 1 tablespoon
- Walnuts -1/2 glass
- Salt - 1/2 teaspoon
- Spices - 1/2 ground coriander, 2 bay leaves, 1 pinch of ground pepper

Preparation:

In a saucepan, heat the oil and fry the coriander and laurel leaves in it. Add spinach and saute for 2-3 minutes. Add bulgur; stirring, frying it until the grains are covered with oil and become transparent. Pour water, cover and cook for 20 minutes. After the nuts are added to the pan, do not stir and cook for another 5 minutes. When bulgur is ready, add the pepper.

Omelet from chickpea flour with tomato

Ingredients:

- Nut flour - 1 glass
- Oat flakes - 0.5 cups of flour
- Ground flax - 2 tablespoons
- Tomato juice - 0,5 glasses
- Water - 0,5 + 1 glass
- Vegetable oil - 2 tablespoons
- Spices: 1 teaspoon black salt, 2 tablespoons dried or fresh herbs
- You can add black pepper, turmeric, dried ginger

- Variations of fillings: paneer, sour cream and greens, spinach, mayonnaise, canned corn, lentil forcemeat with cabbage and carrots

Preparation:

Mix the flax with half a glass of water and set aside for 10 minutes. Combine the oatmeal and chickpea flour, add salt and spices, dried herbs. Stir the tomato juice with 1/2 cup of water and pour into a dry mixture. Add soaked flax and oil, mix well; the dough should turn out thick, like a pancake. Leave to stand for 10-15 minutes to determine if you need to add liquid; if necessary, add more water and mix again. Bake an omelette on a smeared preheated frying pan, over medium heat, about 5-7 minutes on one side and 3-4 on the other. Dough is heavily poured, so you need to distribute it in a frying pan with a fork or spoon; Do not bake bread, just wait until the surface is dry. In principle, at this step you can stop and eat an omelet from the chickpea flour with a juicy vegetable salad. Or, on one half of an omelette put any of the available fillings, cover another and serve at the table.

Vegetables in the oven

Ingredients:

- Eggplant - 1 piece
- Zucchini - 1 piece
- Sweet pepper red - 1 piece
- Sweet pepper yellow - 1 piece
- Sweet pepper green - 1 piece

- Tomato - 3 pieces
- Olive oil - 3 tablespoons
- Balsamic vinegar - 1 tablespoon
- Parsley - 1 beam
- Rosemary - 1/2 teaspoon
- Basil - 1/2 teaspoon
- Thyme - 1/2 teaspoon
- Oregano - 1/2 teaspoon
- Sage - 1/2 teaspoon
- Salt

Preparation:

Wash vegetables, aubergine, zucchini cut into mugs, peppers and tomatoes cut in half. Place the vegetables on a baking tray, sprinkle with oil and sprinkle with spices. Bake at a temperature of 180 C for about 30-40 minutes. Then peppers and tomato to peel and cut into cubes. In a salad bowl, combine the olive oil, balsamic vinegar and finely chopped parsley, then add the vegetables and move.

Stew with tofu

Ingredients:

- Tofu - 200 g
- Carrots - 1 piece
- Zucchini - 1 piece
- Tomato - 1 piece
- Green peas - 100 g
- Tomato paste - 3 tablespoons

- Coriander - 1 teaspoon
- Black pepper - 1 teaspoon
- Curry - 1 teaspoon
- Nutmeg - 1: 2 teaspoon
- Bay leaf - 2 pieces
- Parsley and coriander

Preparation:

Tofu cut into cubes and fry until golden brown. Chop the carrots, tomatoes. Cut the zucchini into large pieces, mix, add bay leaf and spices, mix with tomato paste. Pour 1 cup of boiling water, stew for 10 minutes. Add after 5 minutes chopped greens. When serving, decorate with green peas.

Burger vegan

Ingredients:

- Flour wheat whole-grain - 250 g
- Wheat flour in / s - 250 g
- Baking Powder - 11 g
- Food soda - 1/2 teaspoon
- Lemon acid
- Poppy - 2 tablespoons
- Sesame - 2 tablespoons
- Flax seeds - 2 tablespoons
- Sunflower seeds - 3 tablespoons
- Water

- Boiled chicken noodles - 300 g
- Wheat Flour - 50 g
- Salt
- Curry - 1 tablespoon
- Turmeric - 1/2 teaspoon
- Semolina - 100 g
- Vegetable oil
- Sweet pepper yellow - 1 piece
- Sweet pepper red - 1 piece
- Lettuce - 1 piece
- Cucumber - 1 piece
- Tomato - 1 piece
- Tomato paste - 2 tablespoons
- Oregano - 1/2 teaspoon

Preparation:

1. Mix two kinds of flour, salt, baking powder, soda and citric acid. Add poppy and sesame, stir. Gradually pour in water and knead an elastic, rather dense dough. Leave it to lie for 15 minutes. To make the dough not dry, cover the bowl with the dough lid. Divide the dough into several parts. Form the balls from them. On the table, pour a little poppy and sesame, put the dough bowl on top and flatten it with your hand. So to form all the biscuits. Bake at 250 degrees for 15 minutes in the middle of the oven. Cut ready buns in half along.

2. Pre-soaked for the night chickpeas, boil for half an hour, drain water, chop chickpeas blender. Mix chickpeas with flour, curry and turmeric. Form the

balls, flatten them to shape the cutlets. Roll each cutlet in semolina. Fry in vegetable oil on both sides over a large fire for 2 minutes.

3. For the sauce, mix the tomato paste, oregano and 2 tablespoons of hot water. On the bottom half of the bun, put a lettuce leaf, thinly sliced vegetables, on top of the chickpea cutlet greased with sauce. On top again are the vegetables and the top of the bun.

Chile con

Ingredients:

- Soya pieces - 300 g
- Polba - 100 g
- Beans - 200 g
- Corn - 50 g
- Carrots - 1 piece
- Sweet pepper - 2 pieces
- Tomatoes - 2 pieces
- Tomato juice - 100 ml
- Cocoa - 1 tablespoon
- Chili pepper - 1 piece
- Cumin - 1 teaspoon

- White pepper - 1 teaspoon
- Coriander - 1 teaspoon
- Oregano - 1 teaspoon
- Salt to taste
- Corn chips - 1 pack
- Greens for filing

Preparation:

For the night soak in cold water beans and polbu. Boil beans and polbu can be in one pan for an hour. Soya pieces boil according to the instructions on the package. Carrots, sweet peppers and tomatoes cut into and simmer in a saucepan with a thick bottom for 15 minutes. Then add the beans, crayfish, corn, soy slices and pour it all with tomato juice. Chili pepper is cleaned of seeds, finely chopped and added to vegetables. Be careful with pepper, if you do not like spicy, its amount should be reduced. Add all recommended spices and cocoa. Leave to simmer for 10 minutes. Serve with finely chopped herbs, decorating a bowl of corn chips.

Manti with mushrooms and lentils

Ingredients:

- Flour - 350 g
- Water - 100 ml
- Lentil - 100 g
- Champignons - 200 g
- Vegetable oil - 2 tablespoons
- Salt pepper

Preparation:

1. Flour the flour, add water and a pinch of salt by parts and knead the dough. Wrap it in a food film and give it a "rest" 30 minutes. Lentils should be washed with cold water and cooked. When lentils are cooked, drain excess water.

2. Fry the cut mushrooms in vegetable oil until excess moisture evaporates. At the end, add salt and pepper. Connect the lentils with mushrooms.

3. Dough roll out on a flour-poured table, cut out circles or squares, put a spoon in the middle of the filling and form manta rays. Cooking manti should be in a steamer or mantyshnitsa 20-25 minutes.

The Vegan Velininge

Ingredients:

- Mushrooms - 350 g
- Walnuts - ¼ cup
- Fresh thyme - 2 teaspoons
- Lentil - 2 cups
- Kinoa - 1 glass
- Vegetable broth - ¼ cup
- Celery - ¾ cup
- Bread crumbs - 1 glass
- Thyme - 2 teaspoons
- Sage - 2 teaspoon
- Rosemary - 1 teaspoon
- Basil - 1 teaspoon
- Parsley - 2 tablespoons

- Oregano - ½ teaspoon
- Salt, pepper to taste
- Flax ground - 2 tablespoons
- Dijon mustard - 1 tablespoon
- Eggplant - 1 large
- Mustard - 1 tablespoon
- Vegan dough - 1 pack
- Vegetable oil - 2 tablespoons

Preparation:

1. Mushrooms and walnuts in a blender. Add thyme. Fry in a dry hot frying pan. It will take about 7-10 minutes. When all the water is evaporated, remove from heat. Heat the broth over medium heat in a large non-stick frying pan. Add celery and simmer until soft and

translucent. Add thyme, sage, basil, oregano and simmer for another minute or two. Add a little more vegetable broth if vegetables stick. Remove from heat.

2. Beat 2 tablespoons of flax seeds together with 5 tablespoons of water. Put in the refrigerator for 10 minutes.

3. In a large bowl, knead lentils. Add kino, bread crumbs, parsley, salt, pepper, flax, Dijon mustard. Mix. Add more bread crumbs to glue, if necessary.

4. Clear the eggplant. Cut them into thin long strips. Season with salt and pepper, grease with olive oil, set aside. Now collect the roll. Lay a piece of eggplant diagonally on a polyethylene film. Leave 3 cm from the end of the film. Cover the eggplant with mustard. Put the mushrooms evenly. Put the stuffing and roll the roll, helping

yourself with a film. Tighten the ends. Place in a refrigerator for 15 minutes.

5. Roll out the dough. Put on film. Put the roll on the dough and wrap it with it. Remove excess and wrap ends. Put it in the refrigerator for 15 minutes. Cover with butter and bake in the oven at 180 degrees for 25-30 minutes.

Cabbage rolls

Ingredients:

- Tomatoes - 800 grams of sliced
- Tomato paste - 150 g
- Vegetable broth - 1 glass
- Vegetable oil - 1 tablespoon
- Cabbage cabbage - 1 piece

- Boiled rice - 1/2 cup
- Mixture of dried vegetables
- Seasonings and salt

Preparation:

1. Prepare the sauce. In the pan, pour a little oil and put the crushed tomatoes. It is advisable to preliminarily pass them by boiling water and remove the skin, without it the tomatoes will be tender. Put the rest of the ingredients for a sauce shortly, bring the mixture to a boil, and then simmer at minimum heat for 20 minutes. You should get a gentle, thick mixture. In the end, you can add a little vegan sour cream or cream and mix.

2. Divide the head of cabbage into separate sheets. Heat the water in a large saucepan and place the sheets there. It is necessary to boil them a little, so that they become softer and it was possible to roll them into rolls. But do not digest, otherwise the cabbage rolls will fall apart. Get the leaves out of the water and cool. Mix all the ingredients for the filling, add ¼ cooked tomato sauce so that the filling is not dry.

3. Put it in the center of the sheet and carefully wrap it. Try to put a lot of stuffing. If necessary, you can pin an envelope with a toothpick, and after cooking remove it.

4. Minimize all the cabbage rolls, then put them on the bottom of the pan, starting with the largest and ending with those that are smaller. Fill saucepan with sauce and add vegetable

broth or water. Bring to a boil, and then minimize the heat. Stew about 40 minutes until soft.

Stewed soybean "meat"

Ingredients:

- Soy meat - 55 g
- Soy sauce - 2 tablespoons
- Carrots - 2-3 pieces
- Medium potatoes - 1 piece
- Flour - 2 tablespoons
- Water or vegetable broth - 1 glass

- Homemade tomato paste - 2 tablespoons
- Bay leaf - 2 pieces
- Ground pepper - ¼ teaspoon
- Salt - ¼ teaspoon
- Peas - 1 cup of frozen

Preparation:

Soak the soy meat in hot water and add 1 tablespoon of soy sauce. Drain and set aside. Vegetables peeled and cut. Add the carrots and potatoes to a large saucepan. Add a little water and cook for 5 minutes, stirring constantly. Add flour and cook another minute or two. Add water or broth and tomato paste. Stir and bring to a boil. Add the remaining soy sauce, soy meat, bay leaf, pepper and salt. Stir, cover and simmer for about 20 minutes. Add the frozen peas and cook for another 10 minutes.

Curry with eggplant and chickpeas

Ingredients:

- Eggplant - 1 piece
- Vegetable oil
- Black mustard - 1 teaspoon
- Masala - 2 teaspoons
- Grated ginger - 1 tablespoon
- Salt and other spices - to taste
- Lemon juice - 1/2 pieces

- Boiled chicken noodles - 200-300 g
- String beans - 100 g
- Vegetable broth - 1 l

Preparation:

1. Eggplants chopped, sprinkled with salt and left for a few minutes. Then rinse and dry. Fry until crusted in butter or bake in the oven. In a saucepan, heat 1-2 tablespoons of oil. Add the seeds of black mustard, fry until cod. Add masala and other spices. Then add the ginger and the beans. Lightly fry and broth. Bring to a boil and cook for about 5 minutes. Salt.

2. Add chickpeas and eggplant. Bring to a boil, season with lemon juice and remove from heat. Serve with boiled rice.

Potatoes with mushrooms

Ingredients:

- Potatoes (mini) - 260 g
- Mushrooms (honey agaric) - 150 g
- Oil (olive) - 15 g
- Thyme (fresh) - 2 g
- Parsley (leaf) - 2 g
- Parsley (chopped) - 1 g
- Salt
- Pepper

Preparation:

1. Wash potatoes, cut large tubers.

2. Blanch beads in boiling water for a few minutes so that they do not lose shape.

3. Add the olive oil to the heated frying pan and fry the thyme sprigs in it. In the frying pan add the potatoes and fry until golden brown. Then add honey agaric, salt, pepper, chopped parsley and mix. Fry for a few minutes. Decorate the dish with fresh twigs of thyme and parsley leaves.

Bulgur with green peas

Ingredients:

- Bulgur - 1/2 cup
- Water - 1 glass

- 1/2 pea green peas
- A few branches of greenery - parsley, cilantro, dill
- Olive oil
- Lemon juice - 1-2 tablespoons
- Salt, spices

Preparation:

1. Without washing bulgur, pour it with a glass of boiling water, add a pinch of salt and cook on low heat for 10 minutes under the lid until the bulgur becomes soft and absorbs all the water. A few minutes after the beginning of cooking, stir the bulgur with a fork so that it absorbs water more evenly.

2. On olive oil fry peas, fresh or frozen, for a couple of minutes, remove from heat.

3. Again loosen bulgur with a fork and transfer the peas to it, as well as all the oil that remained at the bottom of the pan. Add chopped greens, season with salt, freshly ground pepper and lemon juice, and then mix well.

Eggplant - steak with celery puree

Ingredients:

- Eggplant - 1 piece
- A couple of slices of stale, boneless bread
- A few sprigs of parsley
- Vegetable oil

- Salt, pepper - to taste
- Celery root - 500 g
- Celery stalk - 1-2 pieces
- Bay leaf - 1 piece
- Olive oil - 50 ml
- Salt
- Nutmeg - 1/4 teaspoon
- Zira - 1/4 teaspoon
- White pepper - 1/4 teaspoon

Preparation:

1. Peel the celery root and cut into cubes. Transfer to a saucepan, add chopped celery cherry and bay leaf, pour water and, boiling, cook for about 20 minutes until soft celery. Drain the water, remove the bay leaf and punch the contents of the pan with a submerged

blender until smooth. Wipe the mashed potatoes through a sieve, season with salt, nutmeg, ground zira and white pepper, after which, gradually adding olive oil, whisk the mashed whisk - this will give it creamy creaminess, and without any cream. Olive oil can be replaced with other vegetable, but certainly delicious, because it plays almost a determining role in the formation of taste mashed potatoes.

2. Cut the eggplant in slanting slices about 1 cm thick, add and set aside. Grind the dried bread together with parsley. Rinse the eggplants under running water, dry with a napkin, season each slice with salt and pepper and oil on both sides, then wrap in breadcrumbs. Bake the eggplant in the oven at 200 degrees for 15 minutes, turning over during cooking.

Chickpeas in tomato sauce

Ingredients:

- Nut - 1 glass
- Rosemary - 2 sprigs
- Bay leaf - 2 pieces
- A few sprigs of parsley
- Lemon - 1/2 pieces
- Tomatoes - 400 g chopped
- Oregano - 1 teaspoon
- Olive oil - 2 tablespoons
- Salt, spices

Preparation:

1. Pour the chickpeas with warm water and leave for 8 hours. After this, drain the water, pour the chickpeas with water again, put on fire and bring to a boil. Boil 5 minutes, then drain again, pour in chickpeas with fresh water, add bay leaf, rosemary and parsley stems, bring to a boil and reduce heat. Boil the chickpeas until soft under the lid with a gentle boil for 1.5 hours.

2. Meanwhile, heat the butter, add the cut tomatoes and reduce the heat. Season the sauce with a pinch of salt, black pepper and dried oregano, and simmer, stirring occasionally and kneading tomatoes with a spatula, about 30 minutes, until a thick and almost uniform consistency.

3. When both chickpeas and sauce are ready, pour the chickpeas together

with the liquid in which it was cooked, to sauce, and simmer over medium heat, occasionally stirring. In the process of mixing, take out the stems and bay leaves from the chickpea and cook for about 20 minutes, or until the sauce becomes the desired consistency. To make the sauce more dense and homogeneous, you can punch a blender about a quarter of chickpeas in a tomato sauce, and then reconnect this thick mass with the prepared dish.

4. Mix in the sauce finely chopped parsley, as well as zest and lemon juice, in the latter being guided by your own taste. Serve chickpeas in tomato sauce, sprinkling it with olive oil and garnishing with finely chopped greens.

Spinach with mushrooms

Ingredients:

- Spinach - 150 g
- Forest mushrooms - 75 g
- Vegetable oil - 2 tablespoons
- A pair of thyme sprigs
- Salt, spices - to taste

Preparation:

1. If you use frozen foods, do not defrost them earlier. Put the frying pan on fire above average, add vegetable oil, warm up and add mushrooms. Fry them for 3-4 minutes, stirring, until golden brown. Add the leaves of thyme, season with

salt and black pepper and fry, continuing to stir, a couple of minutes.

2. Now add the spinach. Periodically stir the contents of the frying pan: to wilting fresh spinach, it takes literally 3-4 minutes, frozen will need a little more.

3. Spinach with mushrooms is well placed on friable rice, couscous, bulgur, kinoa or any other cereal that gratefully perceives the oil draining from it.

Pasta with homemade tomato sauce

Ingredients:

- Pasta - 100 g of durum wheat

- Cherry tomatoes - 5-6 pieces
- Olive oil - 1 tablespoon
- Tomatoes - 100 g
- Carrots - 25 g
- Celery stalk - 10 g
- Salt

Preparation:

1. Boil the pasta.
2. Prepare the sauce: chop carrots and celery, mix with sliced tomatoes without skins. Put on the fire and simmer for about 15 minutes. Add spices and salt. Mix. Remove from heat, cool, pierce in a blender and strain.

3. Cherry tomatoes cut into halves. Put a paste in the plate, pour the sauce, add the tomatoes, olive oil and mix.

Eggplant with coconut milk

Ingredients:

- Eggplant - 1 piece
- Chili pepper - 1 pod
- Cilantro - 1 bundle
- Olive oil - 1 tablespoon
- Coconut milk - 150 ml
- Sesame for decoration
- Salt and pepper

Preparation:

Cut eggplants in large strips. Fry in a large amount of olive oil in a frying pan. Add the finely chopped chilli into the frying pan. After the vegetables are cooked, add the coconut milk and hold on the fire for a few more minutes. Put the vegetables in a bowl and sprinkle with fresh cilantro and sesame seeds.

Vegan Shakshuka

Ingredients:

- Tofu - 90 g

- Pumpkin baked - 20 g
- Flat cake - 1 piece
- Tomatoes - 100 g
- Bulgarian pepper - 80 g
- Olive oil - 1 tablespoon
- A pinch of ground ginger
- Pinch of ground paprika
- Pinch of dry curry mixture
- Bay leaf - 1 piece
- Drinking water - 70 ml
- Fresh greens
- Salt

Preparation:

For the filling, fry in finely chopped tomatoes, pepper along with all the spices and water. Ready-made stuffing put on a plate, make a few grooves, put them in tofu, on top of the pumpkin. Decorate the dish with herbs. Serve with a scone, dried in a toaster or oven.

Pancakes with zucchini and sauce

Ingredients:

- Zucchini - 150 g
- Kinoa - 50 g
- Flour - 20 g
- Fresh or pickled cucumbers - 40 g

- Soya sour cream - 100 g
- Salt, spices

Preparation:

Grate the zucchini on a coarse grater, add pre-boiled cinnamon, form 4 pancakes, roll them in flour, fry on a grill or frying pan on both sides, then bake for 7 minutes in the oven at 180 ° C. For feeding, you can thinly cut the remains of zucchini into slices and dry it on a separate baking dish, like chips. Smaanu and cucumbers mix in a blender to the state of the sauce. Or cucumbers can be finely chopped separately and then mixed with sour cream.

Vegetable stew in Provençal

Ingredients:

- Potatoes - 4-6 pieces
- Bulgarian pepper - 2 pieces
- Eggplant - 1 piece
- Zucchini - 1 piece
- Olives - ½ cans
- Marinated cucumbers, carrots

Preparation:

Boil the potatoes in a peel, bake whole sweet peppers, eggplant, zucchini and then cut them into strips, add to the boiled potatoes. Also add marinated olives and pickled carrots, cucumbers.

Part 2

Introduction

With this book, you will learn how to transition into living vegan or just adding some vegan meals to your diet. Life healthier and enjoy the process. All while helping the environment and yourself feeling better, energized and fit.

Thanks again for downloading this book, I hope you enjoy it!

Step 1: Know the History of the Vegan Movement

The decision to become a vegan should be a result of gathering relevant information about the diet plan and the best way to start it. It is also advisable to trace the roots of the vegetarian and the vegan movement. One can always connect the history of veganism with the history of vegetarianism.

Contrary to popular belief, the idea of vegetarianism started during the sixth century, B.C. The Greek mathematician Pythagoras was actually a vegetarian. Abstaining from meat, according to Pythagoras, was rooted in his spiritual beliefs.

In fact, until 1944, a diet without animal products was called a Pythagorean diet until Donald Watson coined the word vegan. As secretary of the Vegetarian Society in Leicester, Watson firmly believed that vegetarianism needed a reform. He was opposed to vegetarians eating dairy and eggs. In fact, he even read a paper entitled "Should Vegetarians Eat Dairy Produce?" in one of the society's meetings.

In November 1944, Watson and a few of his comrades founded the Vegan Society, a faction group from the Vegetarian Society. It was on the same month that the society's periodical The Vegan News was first published, still being published today as The Vegan.

Following the footsteps of its British predecessor, Jay Dinshah founded the American Vegan Society in 1960. In 1987, a book entitled Diet for A Small Planet by John Robbins documented in a comprehensive way all there is to know about being a vegetarian, debunked the protein myth and exposed the environmental consequences of animal agriculture. This book introduced the term vegan into the vocabulary. In the 1990s, the American Dietetic Association espoused the Food Pyramid that clearly shows the benefits of having lots of grains, vegetables, fruits and beans in one's diet.

The present-day Vegan community around the world involves many organizations and individuals who are all committed to the lifestyle of not exploiting animals. Knowing these facts will help put the decision of becoming a vegan into perspective, knowing that our decision comes from somewhere and has a great history rooted on facts and research.

Step 2: Plan the Shift Into Being a Vegan

One needs to know what being a vegan entails. One thing that one needs to know is that this is a shift in lifestyle and it should be a gradual process. A good thing to do is to devise a plan of action and work within a specific timetable that is comfortable and sustainable for you.

The Academy of Nutrition and Dietetics in America says that a vegan diet is only healthy if it is well-rounded and planned out. One needs to decide when to start on gradually making small changes, and one way of doing that is making a schedule of when to shift into becoming a full-pledged vegan. Since it is a gradual process, one also needs to decide whether to become a vegetarian first, and then gradually shift to becoming a vegan, which many people are actually doing.

A vegetarian diet has plant-based foods. The diet plan does not consist of animal flesh. While there are vegetarians who eat eggs and/or dairy products, others avoid these foods. A vegan diet does not include all animal products and by-products. It is a huge decision, and weaning off food that you've been used to all your life may be difficult, but a careful plan of action should be done to reap its full benefits and motivate you to continue on your path. For instance, make an initial plan to give up one kind of non-vegan food per week, and do it for a month. Then move on from there.

Step 3: Make Small Changes

A great way to start off your vegan plan of action is to ease into it. This will make the choice much easier, if the adjustment is made not abruptly, but gradually. The transition of your body will also be easy. Any sudden, drastic change in your diet will affect your body tremendously, especially changes in being an omnivore to becoming a full-pledged vegan.

One thing to remember is to listen to what your body is telling you and avoid forcing yourself to change everything completely without proper guidance and information. You may start by removing cheese, then eggs, then milk and dairy products, then meat. It is also advisable to remove one type of animal from your diet at a time. One can also start with being vegetarian, then removing eggs and dairy eventually.

The most important thing is to go at your own pace. You may also begin with one thing that you consume the most, and then start substituting with the vegan version.

For instance, if you drink milk every day, you may begin substituting it with almond milk. One great way of doing it is taking into account all the junk food in your home, such as anything with refined flour, sugar and processed food. One may target one type of junk food and start with a healthier vegan option. If you have potato chips and cheese dip, why not have some nacho cheese and salsa. If you like candy, why not eat apples and bananas?

It takes months, even years to build a habit, so a gradual approach is always the better choice. Going cold turkey is like setting yourself up for failure.

Step 4: Do It Right - Learn About Vegan Nutrition

Learning as much as you can about nutrition, especially the nutrition behind vegan food is essential to be able to forge ahead in this path. As people will quiz you on where you get your nutrients if you are vegan, it is good to know that there are several nutrients that one can get from a vegan diet.

First, you should understand that turning to the vegan diet does not mean that you should deprive yourself of protein. Meat, poultry, dairy and eggs are not the only sources of protein. There are several plant-based products that are protein-rich. These include soybeans, tofu, nuts, beans, seeds, chickpeas, mushrooms, broccoli, quinoa and whole grains, and you can include them in your diet.

Cow's milk is not the only source of calcium. It is abundant in kale, broccoli, almonds and collard greens. You can also find it on rice or soymilk and orange juice.

There is a myth that Omega-3 fatty acids only come from fish, but that is not true. Fish actually get omega-3 from their diet, which includes algae. Drinking supplements containing omega 3 derived from algae is recommended. Since it is a fact that our body needs Omega-3 fatty acids for our brain, heart, skin and joint health, we need to look for other sources in our diet. Canola oil, walnuts and flaxseeds are good sources of omega-3.

Vegans have always been stereotyped as anemic and pale, but the fact is the rate of anemia among vegans is more or less similar to the rest of the population. Iron-rich vegan foods include spinach, black-eyed peas, chickpeas, lentils, beans, oatmeal, sunflower seeds, molasses, quinoa and nuts.

Vitamin C aids in the absorption of iron, so consuming foods that are rich in both iron and vitamin C is very beneficial. For instance, eating tomatoes with beans or lentils and broccoli are good pairings. Green leafy vegetables are rich in both iron and vitamin C.

Vitamin B12 is presumed to be found only in animal foods. However, it is also possible to find it in fortified nutritional yeast, soy and rice milk. Vegans are encouraged to take a supplement to get ample amounts of Vitamin B12.

As for iodine, vegans can source them from sea vegetables, iodized salt and some beans. Supplementation is necessary because sea vegetables are hard to come by and most vegans are also controlling their salt intake.

Step 5: Learn as Much as You Can About the Benefits of Being a Vegan

Being a vegan has many benefits. In order to have credible and trustworthy information, it is crucial to research and learn about it. It helps to read books on the subject such as The Original Fast Foods by James and Colleen Simmons, Fit for Life by Harvey and Marilyn Diamond and The China Study by T. Colin Campbell. If you're not a big reader, then watching films like King Corn, Supersize Me, Fast Food Nation, Planeat, Food, Inc. and Forks over Knives is beneficial. There are also numerous websites on the subject.

If done right, a vegan diet can lower cholesterol, reduce diabetes and obesity risk and reduce heart attack risk by 25%. Some other benefits of a vegan diet are the following:

A vegan diet contains no cholesterol and almost zero saturated fat. This prevents heart disease and reduces the risk of cancer. A low-fat vegetarian diet stops the progression of artery disease or prevents it entirely. Animal products can clog arteries, inhibit energy and slow down the immune system. This is because a vegan diet has more fiber and has more antioxidant rich components.

Fruits and vegetables are also full of disease-fighting phytochemicals that boost immunity and prevent a range of illnesses. Eating vegan therefore is healthier. If you live a healthier life, then you also live longer. When one stops eating processed foods and those that are rich in saturated fats, they will keep their weight down. A vegan diet filled with plant-based, fiber-rich fruits and vegetables, and unrefined complex carbohydrates can keep off the weight while keeping the stomach feeling full.

Eating animal-based food products that are laden with cholesterol results in clogged arteries, thus muscles do not get enough oxygen resulting to inability to optimize energy. Since vegans are free of cholesterol-laden, artery-clogging foods, they generate more usable energy. Whole grains, fruits, vegetables and legumes are also high in complex carbohydrates that supply the body with energizing fuel.

Waste excretion, which is essential in our bodily functions, is more regular when we consume vegetables that have more fiber to push waste out of the body. Vegetarians are not prone to constipation and hemorrhoids.

Vegans are also environmental advocates since they only eat mostly what the land produces. In addition, recent discoveries show that the meat industry dumps chemical and animal waste runoff from factory farms into river and streams, causing pollution. These come from confined poultry and cattle farms.

A lot of animal-based products that are commercially sold are laced with steroids and hormones, particularly meat and dairy products. Animals growing in slaughterhouses have diets tainted with antibiotics and other chemicals. Being a vegan means that we can avoid ingesting these toxic chemicals.

Vegans do not contribute to cruelty to animals. Each year, ten billion animals are slaughtered for human consumption. Most animals that are used for food today are factory-formed and didn't roam freely in farms. They are confined to very small stalls their entire lives until they are ready to be slaughtered.

Step 6: Look at the Lives of Other Vegans

It is good to take a look at the lives of people who are vegans in order to seek out role models and for us to realize that we are not alone in our advocacy. Many famous and accomplished people are actually vegans, and they act out as spokespersons for many vegan causes. However, there are also ordinary people living quiet lives who are doing great things for veganism.

The internet is full of these wonderful people, and their stories serve as great encouragement in starting your own vegan lifestyle. Some inspiring celebrity vegans are Ellen DeGeneres, Alanis Morissette, Mike Tyson, Alicia Silverstone and Ben Stiller. There are also ordinary people, not celebrities, whose wonderful vegan journeys are equally inspiring. Their journey towards becoming a vegan, and the reasons why they're doing it will help you jumpstart your own journey and create your own story.

Start It Right

Step 7: Visit a Doctor

Experts recommend that before deciding to go vegan, a complete physical check-up is necessary. Your physician should know that there are certain considerations to take into account once you become a vegan since he or she knows your medical history. Doctors do not oppose to veganism, and a very good doctor will know supplements and substitutes that your body needs in order to maintain all its nutritional requirements.

Your doctor will also be able to shed some light on how to maintain a balanced diet and be able to recommend essential vitamins and minerals that your body needs. A blood test can also help confirm levels of vitamins and trace elements in your body.

It is also a good idea to find a vegan doctor who will be able to give you proper advice not only based on head knowledge and training, but on his personal lifestyle. A good number of doctors advocate veganism, and the main thing for them is to be able to give the patients advice on a vegan diet program that contains high micronutrients and fiber, but low in sugar, fat, calories and salt content.

Step 8: Commit to a Vegan Lifestyle

As much as it is avoiding certain kinds of food in your diet, veganism is a state of mind and a lifestyle. This means that all other aspects of your life are committed to being vegan. Committing to this lifestyle requires you to know and understand your exact reasons for doing this. Ask yourself, is it the fact that you want to be compassionate to animals? Or is it because of your concern for the environmental effects of factory farming? Is it because you want to live a healthy life?

The reason has to be clear to you, so you can also articulate this reason to other people clearly, when they ask or even when they see you. This positive move is a promise to yourself, then to your family, and to the community.

Step 9: Tell Your Family and Close Friends

It is important to let the people in your life, particularly the people you live with, that you are switching to a vegan lifestyle. Your family and closest friends are your support system, and knowing that they understand and are willing to help you with your decision on becoming a vegan is a good encouragement.

While we cannot directly tell them to switch to a vegan lifestyle, we can certainly influence them when they see that we are committed to it. It is important to remember that each one of us have our own journeys. Maybe in the long run, they will see your dedication and make the same decision to become vegans themselves.

As you have this new lifestyle and are learning wonderful things about being a vegan, we are very eager to share this with our loved ones. It is important to remember to have compassion and not to speak in a judgmental and preachy tone. Explaining the importance of your food choices should always be based on love and kindness. One way of expressing that is by cooking a really delicious vegan meal that you can share with your family and friends.

Step 10: Wean Off on Eggs

As a vegan, weaning off on eggs can prove to be a challenge if you like baked goods and enjoy breakfast foods that mostly contain eggs. However, eggs are easy to replace. There are several websites and books that highlight egg substitutes in baking favorite foods.

Since eggs add moisture and leavening to baked goods such as cookies, pastries and cake, egg substitutes have to do the same functions and taste good at the same time. Common egg replacements while baking are applesauce, mashed banana, canned pumpkin or squash. For desserts and sweets, baked pastries and cakes, other egg replacement options aside from the ones mentioned above are soy or coconut yogurt, potato starch, puréed prunes and mashed potatoes. Other plant-based versions serve the function of eggs in savory cooking. Tofu and chickpea flour are both excellent replicators of egg texture and flavor. Vegan scramble, omelet or quiche use chickpea flour or tofu instead of eggs and they are equally delicious.

Step 11: Wean Off on Milk and Dairy

There are several delicious plant-based alternatives to cow's milk. Soy, almond and rice milk are healthy and delicious alternatives. In cooking milk-based products, sweeter dishes can use coconut milk, vanilla almond milk and hazelnut milk.

Soy milk has almost the same nutritional value as dairy milk, minus the fat and cholesterol. Most soy milk brands are also fortified with Vitamin B12. Rice milk does not have the same thick consistency as soy milk, but it is sweet and a good milk substitute for desserts. It is also a great substitute for milk in your morning cereal. Nut-based milks, such as almond and cashew milk have a nutty taste that could be used for non-savory recipes.

As for other dairy products such as cheese and butter, you can find many alternatives in the market. The creamy taste that we look for in dishes such as macaroni and cheese and lasagna can be duplicated with plant-based ingredients. Creamy vegan sauce recipes are abundant and yummy, too.

Step 12: Be Familiar With Vegetables

We all know that vegetables are full of nutrients and have many health benefits. They are particularly excellent sources of vitamin C, beta-carotene, riboflavin, iron, calcium and fiber. Vegetables are available in many varieties including leafy green such as spinach and lettuce, cruciferous such as cabbage, broccoli and cauliflower, marrows such as pumpkin, cucumber and zucchini, roots such as potato and carrots, edible plant stems such as asparagus and celery and alliums such as onions and garlic.

We will also include legumes in this list, though they are not technically vegetables. Legumes are rich in protein. They also aid in digestion and eliminate harmful toxins from our body. Legumes come in the form of soy products such as tofu and soybeans, legume flours such as chickpea, lentil and soy flour, dried beans and peas and fresh beans and peas such as snow peas, green pea, broad beans and butter beans.

Although not technically vegetables, it is also important to note that mushrooms are also important to a vegan diet and will be included in this list. The most important aspect of mushrooms is their umami, meat-like taste. They pack loads of rich, earthy flavor.

Step 13: Research on Vegetable Recipes

Recipes incorporating vegetables for vegans are numerous on the internet. They are all delicious and healthy, and incorporate vegan ingredients.

Eggplant is a popular vegan vegetable, and apart from making parmigiana, it is actually a very versatile and delicious vegetable to cook with. Some great eggplant recipes are eggplant burgers and eggplant fries with marinara dipping sauce.

Potatoes, with their creamy texture, are also popular vegetables for vegans. There a lot of things we can do with potatoes such as baking, boiling and frying. Popular potato dishes are Creamy Potato and Cauliflower Soup, Baked Potato and even Chocolate Potato Cake.

Beans and legumes are best included in hearty soups and stews. They also work best in chili-style dishes. Lentils, on the other hand, have always replaced meat in a lot of dishes since they are hearty. Some known lentil dishes are Lentil Burgers, Lentil Meatballs and Lentil Stew.

Step 14: Know Your Fruits

Water and fresh raw nutrients found in fruits are vital parts of the vegan diet. Fruits have antioxidants and phytonutrients that are beneficial for the healthy functioning of the human body. You can eat fruits either raw or in a form of juice or smoothie. Dried fruits are also great sources of iron plus vitamins and minerals.

Since fruits are relatively accessible and easy to eat, it can be easy to over-eat them, which is not a good thing also. Overeating any type of food can cause stress to our digestive system, and due to its relatively high sugar content, overeating fruit is also not good to our health.

Fruits are categorized as sweet, like bananas, grapes and papaya, acidic like lemons, limes and strawberries, sub-acidic like cherries, mangoes and apples, melons, and high fat like olives and avocado. Some common dried fruits that you can snack on are apricots, raisins, prunes, pineapple, figs, cherries and cranberries.

Step 15: Research on Fruit Recipes

Vegetarian fruit recipes are abundant on the internet and published cookbooks.

Although fruits are equally good when eaten on their own, mixed with herbs, baked, mixed, and fried food are equally good as well. Smoothies are also popular fruit recipes.

Vegan green teas, banana and strawberry smoothies, cashew, mango and blueberry smoothies and honeydew almond milk smoothies are some of the more popular vegan smoothies around. Popular vegan pie recipes are blueberry pie, apple pie, and vegan peach pie. Fruit salsas and fruit salads are great accompaniments to vegan main courses.

Step 16: Look for Other Protein Sources - Soy

Soy is a popular complete protein source. When we say complete protein, it means that it is a source of nine essential amino acids that the body cannot naturally produce. Not only is it rich in protein, it is also packed with calcium, zinc, iron and other nutrients. In fact, soybeans have been proven to reduce cholesterol and prevent prostrate cancer. The most popular soy products are soymilk and tofu. Most new vegans or even vegetarians are wary with tofu, but it does not taste bad if prepared well. Varieties such as tempeh and natto are fermeted soy products, and are both used in vegan cooking as well.

Some ideas on using tofu aside from milk substitutes would be to use it as a salad dressing or spread. Just blend it with garlic, onion and seasoning, and it will taste good! There are many recipes for cooking tofu on the internet and in popular vegan recipe books.

Step 17: Look for Other Proteins Sources Apart From Soy

Complete protein sources should contain the nine essential amino acids in correct proportion to our dietary needs. While most animal-based foods have complete proteins, vegans will not be in danger of protein deficiency with lots of plant-based options.

Aside from soybeans, other complete protein sources are quinoa, buckwheat, chia seeds, beans, lentils and spirulina.

Quinoa originates from the Andes, South America. Not only is it a complete protein, quinoa is also gluten-free and a calcium, phosphorus and iron source. Preparing quinoa is easy; it is usually boiled and simmered in water like rice and couscous.

Buckwheat is a type of grain native to Asia. This gluten-free fruit seed has 9 essential amino acids, along with fiber, iron and zinc. It is widely eaten in the form of noodles in Japanese and Korean dishes. You can also use it in pancakes, rice and porridge.

Chia seeds are also complete protein sources. You can eat them raw or grind them into flour. It is also possible to add them to fruit juices, and in salads and sandwiches. Fiber-rich chia seeds are the richest vegetable sources of essential omega-3 fatty acids. You can store them in the pantry for years without losing their flavor and nutritional value.

Lentils and beans, both part of the legume family, are excellent sources not only of complete proteins, but also of soluble fiber, which helps lower cholesterol levels, and minerals such as iron and zinc.

Spirulina is a dense, freshwater type of algae. One ounce of spirulina has 2 grams of complete protein. You can add the powder to smoothies and use its flour variety to make pasta or bread.

Eating and Cooking Vegan Good

Step 18: Know More About Plant-Based Ethnic Food

There are numerous other plant-based cuisines in the world, and starting your vegan journey means looking into world food cultures and being adventurous. Due in large part to the Buddhist culture, many Asian cuisines are plant-based. There are great dishes in Vietnamese, Thai and Japanese cuisine that highlight vegetables and other plant-based ingredients. Mexican food relies on spice and flavor and an abundance of legumes is a staple in their diet. A Mexican vegan diet can incorporate veggie tacos, fajitas and burritos.

Ethiopian food is also ideal for vegans because they have many spicy soups and stews with legumes and vegetables as their main ingredients. They usually serve this with sourdough flatbreads or bread made from teff flour, which is very nutritious. Indian food is also ideal for vegans because there is an entire cuisine dedicated to vegetables and spices. Due to Hinduism, there are countless plant-based Indian recipes that are delicious and nutritious. Mediterranean food is also great for vegans because there are a various vegetables and legumes that are part of their local cuisine.

Step 19: Look for Vegan Versions of Your Favorite Food

Because we have been used to tasting our favorite dishes from childhood, we do tend to miss them. Vegans do not need to be deprived because there are a lot of remakes of favorite recipes that pack a lot of flavor. Popularly dubbed as "veganizing", there are a lot of popular sources of recipes that turn old non-vegan favorites into vegan favorites.

There are vegan versions of favorite comfort foods such as Macaroni and Cheese that uses butternut squash, "Popcorn Chicken" which uses tofu, spaghetti and "meat" balls, Peanut Butter banana chip cookies and chocolate cupcakes with avocado chocolate icing. There are even vegan versions of burger and pizza.

Classic meat dishes also have vegan versions. Some examples are Vegan Chicken Noodle soup, Vegetable Paella, Vegetarian Pot Pie and Mushroom burgers.

Step 20: Plan Your Vegan Menu

In planning our vegan meals, we need to think about how to do it without being overwhelmed or confused, and at the same time, we need to make sure that we are getting the nutrition that our body needs.

It is always a good idea to start planning for a two-week duration, do your grocery shopping, and proceed from there. The first step is to determine what meals you are planning to have. We usually plan for the three major meals of the day - breakfast, lunch and dinner. However, we also should plant for in-between meal snacks. We should think about the core ingredients for each meal.

For breakfast, we can begin with cereal, oatmeal and soymilk. For lunch and dinner, we can start with simple vegan staples that are easy to cook such as beans and legumes, vegetables and tofu. For snacks, we can consider dried or fresh fruit, nuts and granola bars. We can always start with the basics then get creative as time goes by.

Step 21: Look for Places to Shop for Vegan Ingredients

These days, most groceries have a natural or health-food section, although smaller groceries may have a limited range of vegan items. There are local health food stores and natural food stores that sell harder-to-find items such as tempeh, chia seeds and other soy products. We can always go to health-food chains like Whole Foods and Trader Joe's that usually offer wider vegan selections. There are also a few places online where one can buy special vegan ingredients.

Depending on the area where you live, there are also weekly farmer's markets and produce markets where we can buy directly from the source. Ethnic grocers that sell Asian, Mediterranean, and Middle Eastern ingredients are also located in some cities. They usually sell at a much lower price than natural food stores. Exotic fruits and spices, sauces and other hard-to-find foods are also available in Ethnic groceries.

Step 22: Shop for Vegan Ingredients

It is a lot of fun to shop and expose yourself to new foods and ingredients. Being a vegan means leaving your comfort zone and trying out vegan recipes from all parts of the globe. Exposure to new ingredients is also part of the adventure. Shopping for vegan ingredients for the first time can be overwhelming and confusing, but there are a few guidelines to remember.

Since vegan food has different categories, it is a good idea to zero in on these aisles in the supermarket. First, go to the fruits and vegetables corner of the supermarket. Simply pick the produce that you planned to buy, and browse around for other interesting ingredients that you may use. Next, proceed to the grains and legumes section. This is where you get your grain or legume of choice. In most supermarkets, the bread aisle is usually located beside the grains section. This is where we get our fill of whole-grain bread, bagels, pita bread and tortilla.

The canned food section is where we usually get tomato sauce, olives, and canned beans. After that, we can proceed to the frozen food section where we can get frozen vegetables. Lastly, we can drop by the snacks section where we can buy vegan snacks.. The best thing to remember in grocery shopping is to check the ingredients well and make sure that they contain all pant-based ingredients.

Step 23: Cook and Be Adventurous

Vegans would have to learn to prepare and cook their own food because most prepared foods in the market contain animal-based ingredients. One advantage of cooking vegan food yourself is that you will have a greater connection and a deeper appreciation to the foods you are eating. As you learn basic recipes and get better at it, your family will also learn to appreciate vegan food.

There are various vegan cookbooks and free recipes online to help vegans get started. They usually have accessible and affordable ingredients, but there are also options for special occasions.

Step 24: Take the Right Supplements

Despite taking the necessary steps to have a balanced diet, we may be missing out on a few core nutrients when we prepare our food. It can get easy to eat the same kinds of foods every day, and in the process neglect the proper types of nutrients that we need as vegans.

This is where the idea of taking supplements comes in. A daily multi-vitamin will ensure that we are getting the right amount of nutrients that we need. Some important vitamins that we should incorporate are Vitamin B12 since there are a few sources of this vitamin in vegan food. No adequate Vitamin B12 means that you are at risk of suffering from anemia.

It is a challenge for a vegan to get omega-3 fatty acids because this usually comes from fatty fish. We could take Omega-3 supplements made from flaxseed oil and incorporate plant-based foods rich in omega-3 fatty acids like walnuts, soybeans and olive oil.

Most vegans also take Vitamin D and iodine supplements. Omnivores usually get iodine from dairy products and seafood, but vegans may not get enough because their only source would be sea salt and sea vegetables.

Step 25: Try Out Vegan Restaurants

Being a vegan should not limit you from eating out and enjoying food in restaurants. Restaurants and fast-food places are starting to offer vegan options on their menus. Some vegans make the effort of searching for vegan menus of their favorite restaurants online. If you anticipate that there will be limited options in the restaurant where you are going to, it is always a good idea to eat beforehand.

We should expect that not all restaurants are sensitive to the vegan lifestyle, so we should be in a state of mind where we accept this fact. You can always ask for a comment card and suggest that they add a vegan menu to their offerings.

The good news is vegetarian and vegan restaurants are cropping up all over, and this tells us that more and more people are adapting this lifestyle. There is now a wide range of vegan restaurants that fit every budget and preference.

Step 26: Share Your Lifestyle

Being a vegan evangelist doesn't mean that you have to be preachy about your lifestyle. Through a positive demonstration, you can help others discover this great lifestyle. Treating them to your vegan cooking could be good idea, if you are confident enough to share the recipes that you have learned. If you discover a great vegetarian restaurant, you can always invite your friends there. The one thing we need to remember here is that we should always have a level of respect to the dietary preferences of others, and they will show the same level of respect to our dietary preferences. Influencing others in our own quiet and loving way is the best form of influence.

Step 27: Get Rid of Other Animal-Based Products

Part of incorporating the vegan lifestyle into your entire being is to get rid of animal-based products in your life that are not related to food. For example, if you have leather wallets, shoes and bags and wool coats that you have purchased before turning vegan, it is best to think about whether you should keep them or gradually replace them.

There are many options on how to get rid of animal-based items. Some people have a yard sale or give them away as gifts. Others make the decision to use them until they wear out, and then replace them with non-animal based products. Other people opt to donate them to charity.

Whatever you decide to do, keep in mind you committed to a certain lifestyle and you should always be consistent in your actions. In order to do this, you should have an understanding of the treatment of animals, particularly how they were treated in making a certain fashion item.

Step 28: Join a Support Group

It is always a great feeling to know that you are part of a certain community where you have the same beliefs and the same concerns. Having a vegan support group will greatly help you air out your concerns and worries. You will also be able to gather information on recipes, current research, and the places to buy vegan-friendly items.

It also helps you expand your world as you discover new restaurants, and even new friends. Whether it's a weekly physical meeting or an online group, it is good to talk about and discuss anything vegan-related.

Sustaining the Vegan Lifestyle

Step 29: Keep Learning

Just as you researched on the vegan lifestyle before deciding to commit to it, sustaining a vegan lifestyle is a life-long learning process. Going vegan is also a learning curve, and this decision is a courageous battle to go against the grain. Being curious and teachable along the way will propel you to be more committed to it. Even if veganism has been around since 1944, it is still a fairly new concept to many people. Continuously seeking new knowledge about this lifestyle will give you motivation to continue on this path.

Step 30: Remember Why

There may be days when you seriously begin to doubt whether this lifestyle is for you or not. There may also be days when you miss cheeseburger too much and you think that going vegan is too much hard work. It is always good to remember why you chose this lifestyle in the first place. Going back to the reason why you did this will always keep you grounded and will motivate you to move forward. Maybe you can remind yourself by going to an animal sanctuary or re-reading your favorite book or watching the video that convinced you to adopt this lifestyle.

Step 31: Don't Give Up

If we fall or falter, we can always get back up and move forward. Being tenacious and persistent despite discouragement will give us the fervor and the drive to succeed. As long as we are confident in what we believe in, we should never falter. There will come a time when being vegan is as natural to you as breathing air and until that time comes, remind yourself of the joys of living a vegan lifestyle.

About the Author

Johnie Burder is author of several cookbooks on Vegan diet. He has written research papers on the topic and currently lives in California.

www.ingramcontent.com/pod-product-compliance
Lightning Source LLC
LaVergne TN
LVHW011946070526
838202LV00054B/4827